YOUR KNOWLEDGE HAS VALUE

- We will publish your bachelor's and master's thesis, essays and papers

- Your own eBook and book - sold worldwide in all relevant shops

- Earn money with each sale

Upload your text at www.GRIN.com
and publish for free

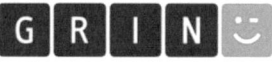

Bibliographic information published by the German National Library:

The German National Library lists this publication in the National Bibliography; detailed bibliographic data are available on the Internet at http://dnb.dnb.de .

This book is copyright material and must not be copied, reproduced, transferred, distributed, leased, licensed or publicly performed or used in any way except as specifically permitted in writing by the publishers, as allowed under the terms and conditions under which it was purchased or as strictly permitted by applicable copyright law. Any unauthorized distribution or use of this text may be a direct infringement of the author s and publisher s rights and those responsible may be liable in law accordingly.

Imprint:

Copyright © 2011 GRIN Verlag
Print and binding: Books on Demand GmbH, Norderstedt Germany
ISBN: 9783668743335

This book at GRIN:

https://www.grin.com/document/431815

Amer Taqa, Nada Z. Mohammed, Alia'a W. Alomari

The Effect of Addition Chlorohexiidine Gluconate (Powder) on the Properties of Heat Cured Acrylic Resin

GRIN Verlag

GRIN - Your knowledge has value

Since its foundation in 1998, GRIN has specialized in publishing academic texts by students, college teachers and other academics as e-book and printed book. The website www.grin.com is an ideal platform for presenting term papers, final papers, scientific essays, dissertations and specialist books.

Visit us on the internet:

http://www.grin.com/

http://www.facebook.com/grincom

http://www.twitter.com/grin_com

The Effect of Addition Chlorohexidine Gluconate (Powder) on the Properties of Heat Cured Acrylic Resin.

ABSTRACT

Aims of the Study: The current study aims to evaluate the effect of the addition of chlorohexidine gluconate (CHX) (powder) on some physical, mechanical properties and antimicrobial effect. **Materials and Methods:** In this study two hundred and forty samples of heat cured acrylic resin (Major base-2) were prepared and divided into: control group(without the addition of CHX) and experimental groups(with the addition of CHX(powder) at (1%, 2%, 3%)) to evaluate transverse strength, tensile strength, , surface hardness, dimensional accuracy, deflection , residual monomer in addition to antimicrobial effect for heat cured acrylic resin before and after the addition of CHX(powder). **Results:** Results showed a statistically significant difference at ($p \leq 0.05$) between control and experimental groups. The addition of CHX (powder) into heat cured acrylic resin increases its flexibility in addition to it's antimicrobial effect. Group of 1% CHX has the highest value of transverse strength, tensile strength ,surface hardness and dimensional accuracy after control group. **Conclusions:** In addition to its antimicrobial effect, CHX increases the flexibility of heat cured acrylic resin. As the concentration of added CHX increased, the flexibility of heat cured acrylic resin specimens will be increased.

Asst Prof Dr **Amer A Taqa** *(BDS, MSc, PhD)* †; *Lect* **Nada Z. Mohammed** *(BDS, MSc)*; *Lect* **Alia'a W. Alomari** *(BDS, MSc)*

الخلاصة

هدف الدراسة: تهدف الدراسة الحالية إلى تقييم تأثير إضافة كلوروهكسيدين كلوكونيت (باودر) على بعض الخواص الفيزيائية والميكانيكية والتأثير المضاد الجرثومي. **المواد وطرق العمل:** في هذه الدراسة تم عمل مائتان واربعون عينة من الراتنج المعالج حراريا (Major base-2) وتم تقسيمها إلى: مجموعة سيطرة (بدون إضافة CHX) وعينات تجربة(مع إضافة CHX بنسب ١%، ٢% و٣%) وذلك لغرض تقيم مقاومة القوة المستعرضة، مقاومة قوة الشد، الصلابة السطحية، دقة وثباتية الحجوم ،الالتواء، البوليمر المتبقي بالإضافة إلى التأثير المضاد الجرثومي للراتينج المعالج حراريا قبل وبعد إضافة CHX(باودر). **النتائج:** أظهرت النتائج وجود اختلاف معنوي عند ($P \leq 0.05$) بين مجاميع السيطرة ومجاميع التجربة . إضافة CHX(باودر) إلى الراتنج الاكريلي المعالج حراريا أدى إلى زيادة مرونته بالإضافة إلى تأثيره المضاد الجرثومي .تمتلك مجاميع التجربة(١%) CHX أعلى قيم لمقاومة القوة المستعرضة، مقاومة قوة الشد، الصلابة السطحية ودقة وثباتية الحجوم بعد مجاميع السيطرة . **الاستنتاجات:** بالإضافة إلى التأثير المضاد الجرثومي ، CHX زاد من مرونة الراتنج الاكريلي المعالج حراريا ، كلما زاد تركيز CHX المضاف زادت مرونة عينات الراتنج الاكريلي المعالج حراريا

Department of Prosthetic Dentistry, †Department of Dental Basic Science, Dentistry College, Mosul University

Key Words: CHX, acrylic resin, flexibility.

Acrylic resin were introduced as a denture base material in 1937[1,2]. In spite of the several limitations of this material, it still remains the most popular material of choice [3-5]. Many studies had been introduced for modification of this material to be more flexible, comfortable, less susceptible to fracture and more acceptable by the patient[6-14].

chlorohexidine gluconate (powder) (CHX) is the most intensely researched preventive agent in dentistry[15],it has been introduced since 1969, it has antimicrobial effect against gram positive, gram negative, yeast and facultative aerobic and anaerobic flora in addition to limited vircucidal effect[16-18]. It has been used as a disinfectant solution[19-22], root canal irrigant [23], treatment of denture stomatitis[24], mouthwash [25], it also can be incorporated into periodontal dressing [26]. Several research has been introduced to study the topical, sustained-release form of CHX by using of a sustained-delivery system of CHX which was applied directly to dental appliances, such a dosage form would be capable to release CHX at low therapeutic level over a long period of time and thus would be effective in the prevention of plaque formation and prevent the side effect of CHX(better test and tooth staining)[27-32].

MATERIALS AND METHODS

Two hundred and forty samples of heat cured acrylic resin (Major base 2) were prepared and divided into:
- ❖ Control group: 60 samples of heat cured acrylic resin without the addition of CHX.
- ❖ Experimental group :180 samples of heat cured acrylic resin with the addition of CHX at (1%, 2%, 3%).

Acrylic resin specimens were prepared in a mold made by investing a hard elastic foil for specific dimensions (according to each test as mentioned bellow) in dental stone that were mixed in a water/powder ratio of 32gm/100ml and placed in the lower half of the flask, then glass slab was placed against the first half till the stone set. After final setting of stone, a conventional flashing procedure was used for the preparation of acrylic resin samples[33].

Acrylic resin samples were mixed and manipulated according to manufacturer directions. Cure was taken to avoid porosities due to entrapment of air bubbles. Trail closure was performed. The specimens were cured in water path with conventional curing cycle, the specimens processed at 74°C for 90 minutes, then the temperature of water path raised to boiling 100°C for 30 minutes(according to manufacture instructions). The samples left for bench cooling for 30 minutes then it finished using tungsten drill and sand paper at low speed [34]. All samples used in this study were evaluated for the presence of porosity by examining them under reflecting light microscope(LOMO Micmed 2) before being tested [6, 35, 36]. After that the samples stored in distilled water at 37°C for two periods of time (2days and 7 days), then the following tests were done to evaluate:

1. Evaluation of transverse strength and deflection : The samples of this test were prepared in dimensions of 65*10*2.5±0.03mm(length, width and thickness respectively)[37]. The test was done by using a 3 points bending on an Instron universal machine(Wolpert, Germany). The samples were deflected until failure occurred. The transverse strength was calculated using the following equation:

Transverse strength$(N/mm^2)=3/2 \times PI \times bd^2$ [38]

b: the sample width (mm) d: the sample thickness(mm)
I: the span length(mm) P: the peak load(N)

The deflection was calculated by using digital vernia in accuracy of 0.001mm Figure(1).
2. Evaluation of tensile strength: The samples of this test were prepared with dimensions of 90*10*3±0.03 mm(length, width and thickness respectively). The tensile strength was evaluated by using Terco universal testing machine. The amount of force applied was 0.1 KN /sec. The results were recorded from a special program on computer of tensile machine for each sample [7].
3. Evaluation of surface hardness test: The samples of this test were prepared with dimensions of 30*15*3±0.03 mm(length, width and thickness respectively). The polished surface was tested for hardness at five different locations then the mean is taken for each surface by using Rockwell hardness tester with an indenter in the form of round steel ball (6.359mm in diameter). The sample was first subjected to a fixed minor load of 10Kg, then load of 50Kg was applied to the sample and the Rockwell hardness number was recorded after application of this load by 15 sec [39].
4. Evaluation of dimensional accuracy: The samples of this test were prepared in dimensions of 65*10*2.5±0.03mm(length, width and thickness respectively) in which their volume standard is equal 1625mm [37],measurement on three dimensions were done by using digital caliper accuracy of 0.001mm [6,7].
5. Evaluation of residual monomer: The samples of this test were prepared with dimensions of 20*20*3±0.03 mm(length, width and thickness respectively) [36]. The samples immersed in distilled water in sealed glass container, then the collected supernated medium was monitored using quartiz cell ultraviolet visible spectrophotometer (CECIL 2000) (λ=254nm) compared with pure monomer. A standard linear calibration curve of methyl methacrylate concentration as a function of absorbency at 254nm was obtained using MMA standard aqueous solution ranged 0.005-0.125ggm/ml[40]. The results were expressed as a percentage of released residual monomer mass with respect to weight of special means [41&42].
6. Evaluation of antimicrobial effect: The samples of this test were prepared as filter disc of (6mm in diameter), the ability CHX to inhibit bacterial growth in vitro was estimated by Disk-Diffusion test[43]. Nutrient agar was used, primary culture was prepared by taking a swap from oral cavity by using sterile loop to test tube contain normal saline. After complete incubation, measuring the inhibition zone around the disc was done to determine the antimicrobial effect.

RESULLTS

Analysis of the mean, standard deviation and Duncan's multiple comparison test showed that the experimental group of 1% CHX has the highest value of transverse strength, tensile strength, surface hardness and dimensional accuracy after control group for 2 and 7 days period Tables(1-4) .While experimental group of 3% CHX showed the lowest value of transverse strength, tensile strength, hardness and dimensional accuracy than control group after 2 and 7 days.

Duncan's multiple comparison test have shown statistically significant difference between control and experimental groups in transverse strength, tensile strength and surface hardness after 2 and 7 days(at $p \leq 0.05$) Tables(1-3). While for dimensional accuracy; Duncan's multiple comparison test Table(4) Showed that there was a statically significant difference between control and experimental groups except that there was no statistically significant difference in dimensional accuracy between control and experimental group of 1%CHX after 2 and 7 days and between experimental groups of 2% CHX and 3% CHX after 7 days at ($p \leq 0.05$). One way analysis of variance Tables(5-8) revealed that there was a statistically significant difference in transverse strength, tensile strength, surface hardness and dimensional accuracy between control and experimental groups after 2 and 7 days at ($p \leq 0.05$).

Table (1): Mean, Standard Deviation and DRMT for the effect of CHX on Transverse Strength of Heat Cured Acrylic Resin

sample	After 2 days			After 7 days		
	Mean(N/mm^2)	SD	DMRT	Mean(N/mm^2)	SD	DMRT
control	94	0.015	A	91	0.077	A
1%CHX	22	0.094	B	25	0.074	B
2%CHX	20	0.060	B	23	0.037	C
3%CHX	15	0.058	C	19	0.083	C

Table (2) Mean, Standard Deviation and DRMT for the Effect of CHX on Tensile Strength of Heat Cured Acrylic Resin

sample	After 2 days			After 7 days		
	Mean(N/mm^2)	SD	DMRT	Mean(N/mm^2)	SD	DMRT
control	56.9	0.054	A	54	0.041	A
1% CHX	39.6	0.035	B	43.6	0.084	B
2%CHX	24.5	0.014	B	26.8	0.073	B
3%CHX	20.1	0.016	C	22.8	0.016	C

Table (3) Mean, Standard Deviation and DRMT for the Effect of CHX on Surface Hardness of Heat Cured Acrylic Resin

sample	After 2 days			After 7 days		
	Mean	SD	DMRT	mean	SD	DMRT
control	110	0.051	A	104	0.0531	A
1% CHX	69	0.051	B	63	0.018	B
2%CHX	67	0.050	B	60	0.051	B
3%CHX	60	0.014	B	55	0.0146	B

Table (4) Mean, Standard Deviation and DRMT for the Effect of CHX on Dimensional Accuracy of Heat Cured Acrylic Resin

sample	After 2 days			After 7 days		
	Mean	*SD*	DMRT	*Mean*	*SD*	DMRT
control	11624.890	0.01	A	11624.86	0.04	A
1% CHX	11624.84	0.01	A	11624.83	0.01	A
2% CHX	11624.61	0.04	B	11624.40	0.01	B
3% CHX	11624.39	0.03	C	11624.18	0.07	B

Table (5): One Way ANOVA of the effect of CHX on Transverse Strength of Heat Cured AcrylicResin

	After 2 days			After 7 days		
S.O.V	DF	MS	F*	DF	MS	F*
Factor	3	7101.1	482.1	3	6231.1	21.3E04
Error	16	1.46		16		
Total	19			19		

*Statistically Significant at $p \leq 0.05$

Table (6): One Way ANOVA of Effect of CHX on Tensile Strength of Heat Cured Acrylic Resin

	After 2 days			After 7 days		
S.O.V	DF	MS	F*	DF	MS	F*
Factor	3	3.067	487.1	3	8.3053	817.9
Error	16	0.039		16	0.0102	
Total	19			19		

*Statistically Significant at $p \leq 0.05$

Table (7): One Way ANOVA of the Effect of CHX on Surface Hardness of Heat Cured Acrylic Resin

	After 2 days			After 7 days		
S.O.V	DF	MS	F*	DF	MS	F*
Factor	3	2421	52.18	3	1912.	31.35
Error	16	77.2		16	36.6	
Total	19			19		

*Statistically Significant at $p \leq 0.05$

Table (8): One Way ANOVA of the Effect of CHX on Dimensional Accuracy f Heat Cured Acrylic Resin

	After 2 days			After 7 days		
S.O.V	DF	MS	F*	DF	MS	F*
Factor	3	0.1878	14.03	3	0.3825	24.78
Error	16	0.0467		16	0.154	
Total	19			19		

*Statistically Significant at p≤0.05

The result in Table(9) showed that there was increase in the deflection of the experimental groups with increasing of the concentration of added CHX. One way analysis of variance Table (10) revealed a statistically significant difference among experimental groups at (p≤0.05).

The experimental group of 1% CHX showed the lowest value of residual monomer release after 2 and 7 days Table(11). One way analysis of variance revealed that there was no statistically significance between control and experimental groups at (p≤0.05) in residual monomer release after 2 and 7 days Table(12).

The results of this study showed that the control group demonstrates the lower change in transverse strength, tensile strength, surface hardness, dimensional accuracy Tables(1-4) and residual monomer release Table(11) from the period of 2 days to 7 days. While the groups with 3% CHX shows the highest change in the values of these tests from the period of 2 days to 7 days.

The antimicrobial test Figure(2) showed that experimental groups of (1%,2% and 3%)CHX have inhibition zone against microorganism of oral cavity.

Table (9) Mean, Standard Deviation and DRMT for the Effect of CHX on Deflection of Heat Cured Acrylic Resin

sample	After 2 days			After 7 days		
	Mean(mm)	SD	DMRT	mean(mm)	SD	DMRT
control	--	------		--	------	
1%CHX	7	0.015	A	6	0.028	A
2%CHX	10	0.01	B	9	0.059	B
3%CHX	12	0.03	C	10	0.021	C

Table (10): One Way ANOVA of the Effect of CHX on Deflection of Heat Cured Acrylic Resin

	After 2 days			After 7 days		
S.O.V	DF	MS	F*	DF	MS	F*
Factor	2	28.764	556.74	3	21.39	134.8
Error	12	0.051		16	0.159	
Total	19			19		

*Statistically Significant at p≤0.05

Table (11) Mean, Standard Deviation and DRMT for the Effect of CHX on Residual Monomer Release of Heat Cured Acrylic Resin

sample	After 2 days			After 7 days		
	Mean(w/w)	SD	DMRT	mean (w/w)	SD	DMRT
control	1.060	0.03	A	0.015	0.01	A
1%CHX	1.046	0.01	A	0.005	0.02	A
2%CHX	1.175	0.05	A	0.047	0.01	A
3%CHX	1.270	0.02	A	0.048	0.02	A

Table (12): One Way ANOVA of the Effect of CHX on Residual Monomer Release of Heat Cured Acrylic Resin

S.O.V	After 2 days			After 7 days		
	DF	MS	F*	DF	MS	F*
Factor	3	0.057	3.69	3	239	1.00
Error	16	0.0155		16	238	
Total	19			19		

*Statistically Significant at p≤0.05

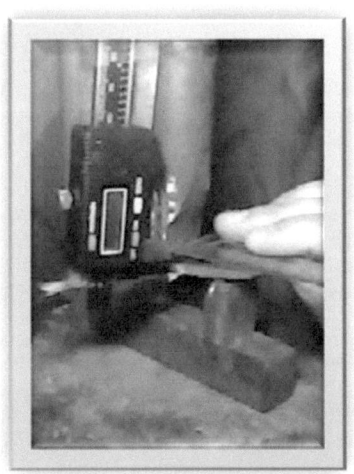

Figure (1): Measuring of the deflection .

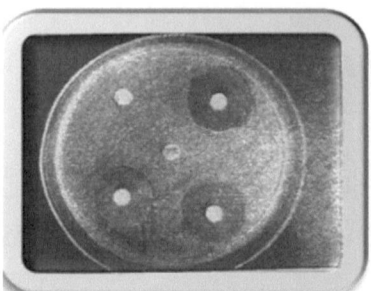

Figure (2): Antimicrobial test of CHX.

DISCUSSION

According to the result of this study the properties of heat cured acrylic resin would be changed after the addition of CHX. This can be explained by the change of the matrix of polymer lattice during polymerization process[44]. However, this do not negate the carriage of CHX in this material(acrylic resin) within oral cavity[31,32] and improvement of flexibility of acrylic resin.

The results of this study Tables(1-3) showed increase in transverse strength, tensile strength and surface hardness of experimental groups after 7 days as compared with that after 2 days period, this can be explained by slow release of CHX from acrylic resin that causes the loss of softness properties and to increase in the rigidity of resin after 7 days[7]. This was in agreement with Naik(2005)[44].

The experimental groups of CHX have shown increase in the deflection Table(9) with increasing the concentration of added CHX, that means increase in the flexibility of the heat cured acrylic resin. The addition of CHX into acrylic resin leads to distribution of the particles of CHX (powder) through the lattice of polymer during polymerization process and this lead to formation of gabs inside polymer lattice, This gab works as a lubricant joints in the polymer lattice [45], thereby increasing the flexibility of experimental groups.

Table (11) showed that the residual monomer release of control and experimental groups after 7 days less than after 2 days. This decrease occurred as a result of the diffusion of the monomer into water and by continues polymerization promoted by the active radicals found in the polymer chains [41, 46]. This table also showed that the experimental sample of 1% CHX has the lowest value of residual monomer release after 2 and 7 days, which could explain the highest value of transverse strength, tensile strength, surface hardness and dimensional accuracy after that of control group as compared with that of experimental groups of 2 % and 3% CHX which show obvious change in these properties Tables(1-4), high level of residual monomer and absorbed water molecules adversely affect acrylic resin properties[13,47,48].

The result of antimicrobial test showed that CHX (powder) has antimicrobial activity after being added to heat cured acrylic resin. This was in agreement with Thaw et al,1981, Ayzkind et al, 1990 and Lamb and Martin,1983, which indicate that CHX(powder) when added to heat cured acrylic resin did not loss the antimicrobial effect.

CONCLUSIONS

In addition to it's antimicrobial effect; the addition of CHX into heat cured acrylic resin increases its flexibility and as the concentration of added CHX increased ; the flexibility of acrylic specimens would be increased.

REFERENCES
1. Craig RG and Power JM. Restorative Dental Material. 10th ed.St Louis, Mosby. 1997: 500.
2. Stafford GD, Bates JF, Huggett R and Handly RW. A Review of the Properties of Some Denture base Polymers. *J Dent*. 1980;8(4) :292-306.
3. Kedjarune U, charoenworaluk N and Koontongkaew A. Release of Methylmethacrylate from Heat-cured and Autopolymerized Resin Cytotoxicity Testing Related to Residual Monomer. *Aust. Dent. J.* 1999;1: 25-30.
4. Cunningham JL. Shear Bond Strength of Resin Teeth to Heat-Cued and High-Cured Denture Base Resin . *J. oral Rehabil.* 2000 ;27:312-316.
5. Jagger DC, Jagger RG, Allen SM and Harrison A. An Investigation into the Transverse Strength and Impact Strength of High Strength Denture Base Acrylic Resin. *J.Oral.Rehabil.* 2002;29:263-267.
6. Amer A.Taqa,Nadira H.,Wafa Abas and Arjwan M Shuker, The Effect of Thyme and Nigella Oil on Some Properties of Acrylic Resin Denture Base, Rafidain dental Journal,2010, Vol.10, No.2,pp.205-213.
7. Amer Taqa; Mohmood Y. and T.K.Bashi, Chemical and Microbiological study of incorporated compounds in denture Base materials, Al-Rafidain Dent.J.,2002, Vol.2, special issue,pp.432-434.
8. Amer A.Taqa,Nadira H. & Radwan H., Evaluation of the effect of curing techniques on color property of acrylic resins, Rafidain Dent. J., 2005, Vol.4, no.1,pp.28-33.
9. Pfieffer P and Rosenbauer EU. Residual Methyl Methacrylate Monomer, Water Sorption and Water Solubility of Hypoallergenic Denture Base Material. *J. Prosthet. Dent.* 2004;92:72-78.
10. Miettinen VM, Vallittu PK. Water Sorption and Solubility of Glass Fiber- Reinforced Polymethy lmethacrylate Resin, *J. Prosthet. Dent.*1996;76:531-540.
11. Machado AL, Vergani CE, Giampaolo ET, Da Slveria MC. Water Sorption, Solubility and Bond Strength of Two Auto Polymerizing Acrylic Resin and One Heat-Polymerizing acrylic resin. J.*Prosthet. Dent.* 1998;80:434-438.
12. Arima T, Murata H and Hamada T. Properties of Highly Cross-Linked Auto Polymerizing Reline Acrylic Resins . *J. Prosthet. Dent.* 1995 ;75:55-59.
13. Takahashi M, Chai I and Kawaguchi R. Effect of Water Sorption on the Resistance to Plastic Deformation of Denture Base Material Relined with Four Different Denture Reline Material. *International Journal of Prosthodontics.* 1998;11(1): 49-54.
14. Jagger D, Harrison A, Vowles R and Jagger R. the Effect of the Addition of Surface Treated Chopped and Continuous Poly(methyl methacrylate) Fibers on Some Properties of Acrylic Resin. *J.Oral Rehabil.* 2001;28(9):865-872.
15. Fardal 0. and Turnbull RS. A Review of the Literatu IC on Use of Chlorhexidine in Dentistry, *J Am Dent Assoc.* 1986; 112: 863-869.
16. Hennessey D. Antibacterial Properties of Hibitane. *J.Clinic. Perio.*1977;4:36-84.
17. Berstein D. In Vitro Virucial Effectiveness of 0.2% Chlorohexidine Gluconate Mouth Rinse. *J.Dent.Res.*1990;69:874-876.
18. Emilson CG. Susceptibility of Various Microorganisms to Chlorohehxidine. *Scand. J. Dent.Res.*1997;85: 255-265.
19. Jalili SN, Abdul Rahim KK and Al-Najjar AR. The Effect of Chlorohexidine Disinfection of Alginate Impression and Dental Stone Cast. *Iraqi Dent. J.*1996;8(1):5-13.
20. Taha MY, Abdul Rahman A and Zakariy NA. Chemical and Microbiological Study of Incorporated Chlorhexidine in Alginate and Stone. *Iraqi. Dent.J.* 2000;25:281-291.
21. El-Ameer SS. The Effect of Long-Term Chlorhexidine Disinfection on the Staining of Acrylic Resin . *Iraqi Dent. J.* 2000;25:145-156.
22. Salem SA, Diha AD and Subhi M. Effect of Chemical Disinfectant on Surface Morphology and Indentation Hardness of Acrylic Resin Cured by Different Methods. *Iraqi Dent. J.*2000;25:21-36.
23. Mohammadi Z and Shariari S. Residual Anti bacterial Activity of Chlorohexidine and MTAD in Human Root Dentine in Vitro. *J. Oral Science.*2008;50(1):63-67.
24. Budtz-Jorgensen E. Hibitane in the Treatment of Oral Candidacies. *J. Clinic. Perio.* 1977;4:117-128.

25. O'Nell TCA. The Use of Chlorohexidine Mouthwash in the Control of Gingival Inflammation . *Brit. Dent. J.*1976;141:276-280.
26. Addy M and Douglas W H. A Chlorhexidine-Containing Methacrylic Gel as a Periodontal Dressing. *J. Periodontal*, 1975; 46: 465-468.
27. Thaw M, Addy M and Handly R. The effect of Drug and Water Incorporation Upon Some Physical Properties of Cold cured acrylic. *J. Biomed Mater Res.*1981;15(1):29-36.
28. Addy M. and Handly R. The Effects of the Incorporation of Chlorohexidine Acetate on Some Physical Properties of Polymerized and Plasticized Acrylics. *J. Oral Rehabil.* 1981; 8(2: 155-163.
29. Zyskind D., Steinberg D, Stabholz A and Friedman M. and Sela MN. The Effect of Sustained Release Application of Chlorhexidine on Salivary Levels of Streptococcus *Mutans* in Partial Denture Wearers. *J. Oral Rehabil.* 1990;17(1):61-66.
30. Lamb DJ and Martin MV. An In Vitro and In Vivo Study of the Effect of Incorporation of Chlorohexidine into Autopolymerizing Acrylic Resin Plates upon the Growth of Candida Albicans. *J Biomaterials.* 1983;4(3): 205-209.
31. Friedmn M, Harari D, Raz H, Golomb G and Brayer L. Plaque Inhibition by Sustained Release of Chlorhexidine from Removable Appliances. *J. Dent. Res.* 1985;64(11): 1319-1321.
32. Mirth DB, Bartkewicz A, Shern RJ and Little WA. Development and in Vitro Evaluation of an Intra-Oral Controlled-Release Delivery System for Chlorhexidine. *J. Dent. Res.* 1989; 68(8):1285-1288.
33. Vallittu PK. Unpolymerized Surface Layer of Autopolymerized Polymethayl methacrylate Resin. *J.oral Rehabil.* 1999;3:208-212.
34. Yannikalis S, Zissis A and Andreopoulos. Evaluation of Porosity in Microwave Processed Acrylic Resin Using a Photographic Method. *J. Prosthet. Dent.*2002;87:613-619.
35. Al-Doori DII. Polymerization of Polymethylmethacrylate Denture Base Materials by Microwave Energy. M.Sc. Thesis 1987, University of Wales, College of Medicine.
36. Hasan RH. Denture Teeth Bond Strength to Heat Water Bath and Microwave Cured Acrylic Resin Denture Base Material (a Comparative Study). M.Sc.2002,University of Mosul, College of Dentistry.
37. American Dental Association Specification Guide to dental materials and device. 1974-1975, pp: 86-96,255-260.
38. Craig R. Restorative Dental Materials. 10th ed. Mosby. St Lauis,1997, pp: 500-551.
39. Isaac RG. Some Properties of Acrylic Denture Base Materials Processed by Two Different Techniques (a Comparative Study) M.Sc. Thesis 1992,University of Baghadad, Colledge of dentistry.
40. Azzarri MJ. Cortize MS, Alesssandrini JL. Effect of the Curing Condition on the Properties of an Acrylic Denture Base Resin, Microwave Polymerized .*J. Dent.* 2003;31: 463-468.
41. DeOliveria MB, LE'on LT, DeL be;cury AA and Consani S. Influence of Number and Position of Flasks in the Monomer Release, Knoop Hardness and Porosity of a Microwave Cured Acrylic Resin. *J. Oral Rehabil.*2003;30: 1104-1108.
42. Sadoon MM. Evaluation of Repairing the Acrylic Denture Base by Using Different, Design and Techniques. M.Sc. Thesis, 2005, University of Mosul, Colledge of Dentistry.
43. Cruicshank R. Medical Microbiology. 12th ed., Churchill Lingstone. Edinburgh, London and Newyork, 1975:169.
44. Naik NV and Jabad JL.Comparision of Tensile bond Strength of Rwsilient Soft Liners to Denture Base Resin. *J. Ind. Prosthet.* 2005;5(2):234-239.
45. Mohammed KA. Polymer Chemistry. 1ST ed. Mosul University, 1993,p: 328.
46. Bartoloni JA, Murchison DF, Wofford DT and Sarkar NK. Degree of Conversion of Denture Base Materials for Varied Polymerization Technique. *J. Oral Rehabil.*2000;27:488-491.
47. Debby MS, Wong ED, Leo YY and Dark ED. Effect of Processing Method on the Dimensional Accuracy and Water Sorption of Acrylic Resin Denture.*.J.Prosthet.Dent.*1999;81:300-404.
48. Sadoon M, Mohammed NZ and AL-Omary A. Residual monomer and Transverse Strength Evaluation of Autopolymerized Acrylic Resin with Different Polymerization Treatment. *AL-Rafidian Dent.J.*2007;7:30-34.

YOUR KNOWLEDGE HAS VALUE

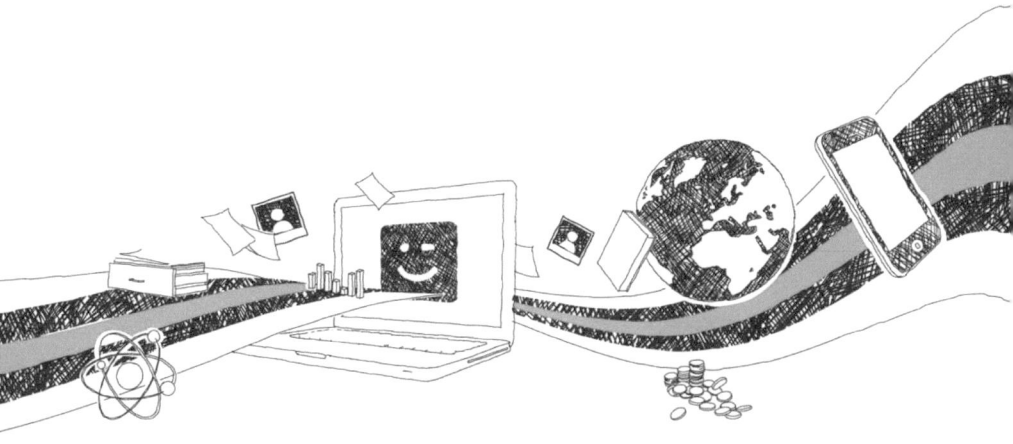

- We will publish your bachelor's and master's thesis, essays and papers

- Your own eBook and book - sold worldwide in all relevant shops

- Earn money with each sale

Upload your text at www.GRIN.com
and publish for free

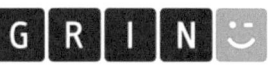